365

ways to be SLIMMER

365 WAYS TO BE SLIMMER

Copyright © Summersdale Publishers Ltd, 2019

Text by Katherine Bebo

An Hachette UK Company
www.hachette.co.uk

Vie Books, an imprint of Summersdale Publishers Ltd
Part of Octopus Publishing Group Limited
Carmelite House
50 Victoria Embankment
LONDON
EC4Y 0DZ
UK

www.summersdale.com

Printed and bound in the Czech Republic

ISBN: 978-1-78685-757-6

Substantial discounts on bulk quantities of Summersdale books are available to corporations, professional associations and othe[?]
organisations. For details contact general enquiries: telephone: +44 (0) 1243 771107 or email: enquiries@summersdale.com.

Neither the author nor the publisher can be held responsible for any loss or claim arising out of the use, or misuse, of the suggestions made
herein. Consult your doctor before making changes to your diet.

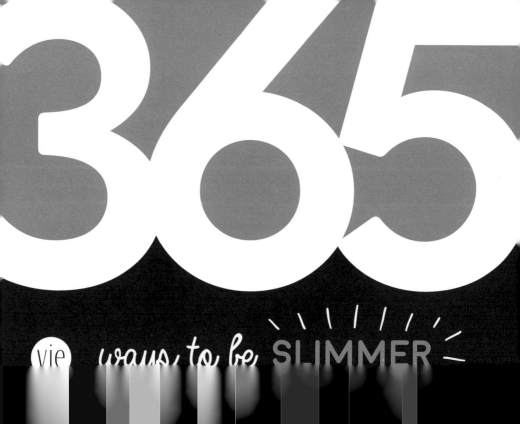

365

vie ways to be SLIMMER

1 You're not responsible for everything that happens to you in life but you *are* responsible for what you put into your body.

2 Ask yourself why you want to be slimmer. Perhaps you want to fit into your old clothes, or you want to form healthy habits. When you understand your motivation, you're more likely to stick to your plan.

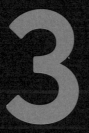

3 Know that food is not your enemy – it's fuel that helps your body perform at its best and it makes you feel your best too!

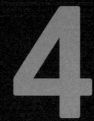

4 You do not need to cut out any food groups from your diet to maintain a healthy weight. Your body needs protein, carbohydrates, fruit, vegetables, sugars and fats – the key is moderation.

You don't need to cut out treats either. As long as you have smaller portions you can still enjoy all your favourite things.

Slimming is not just about eating the right food: it's vital to factor exercise into your routine as well.

7

Losing weight successfully is largely down to your mindset, so feed your mind as well as your body with things that make it strong. Pick out a few positive mantras to help keep you motivated and feeling good. Repeat them to yourself whenever you need a boost.

Small steps lead to big changes.

9 I will be the healthiest version of myself.

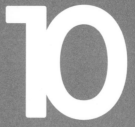

10 I will nourish myself and I will flourish.

11 Food is fuel.

I am getting stronger every day.

I cannot change yesterday,
but I can change today.

Take it one day at a time.

There's no way around it: losing weight in a healthy, sustainable way is a slow process. If you have patience and remain consistent, you will see results.

Be wary of fad diets, or anything that sounds too good to be true. There are no shortcuts when it comes to your health.

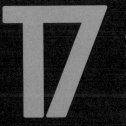

17

Crash diets might appear to be a quick-win slimming solution, but be aware that they do more harm than good in the long term.

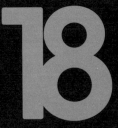

18

If you suddenly reduce your calorie intake, your body's starvation mode is triggered. Your metabolism slows down to conserve energy, so you will be burning fewer calories than normal. Your body will also work hard to store fat rather than lose it – which is the opposite of what you want.

19

Extreme diets which involve depriving the body of calories can also weaken your immune system and lead to serious heart problems, because you'll be missing out on vital nutrients that your body needs such as protein, calcium and iron.

20

Grehlin, often called the 'hunger hormone' is what makes us feel hungry and stimulates our appetite. When your body is being starved, the levels of this hormone are increased, so you feel hungrier and want to eat more than normal.

21

If your body and mind are in an energy-deprived state, it's much harder for you to ignore cravings for unhealthy, processed foods, and to resist the urge to binge eat.

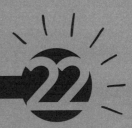

Crash dieting won't give you that healthy feel-good glow. Your energy levels drop when you don't fuel your body properly, leading to physical and mental exhaustion, light-headedness and nausea. It's even thought that it can affect your brain activity, making you feel low and irritable.

23

Of the weight that you do lose while on a crash diet, a portion of that is likely to be muscle rather than fat. Once you come off the diet, the first thing the body will do is replenish its fat stores. So, even if you do lose weight in the short-term, you will have lost muscle and are likely to gain back fat in its place.

24

In contrast, when you lose weight slowly in a controlled and sustainable way, your metabolism remains steady, your muscle mass remains consistent (or increases), your hormone levels stay balanced and your body and mind are healthy.

25

If you feel yourself being tempted by the thought of a drastic diet, remind yourself that your body is an incredible and complex thing, and it needs the right fuel to be at its best to keep you happy and healthy.

26

Instead of thinking 'I have to eat healthily', think 'I want to eat healthily'. This helps to put you in a positive and motivated frame of mind.

27

Think of slimming as a marathon, not a sprint.

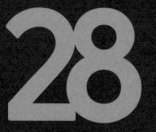

28

Write down your favourite inspiring statement and put it somewhere you will see it. It will remind you of your goals and keep you motivated.

Choose an inspiring photo and put it on your fridge, or in the place where you keep your snacks – perhaps a photo of a celebrity with a healthy figure you admire.

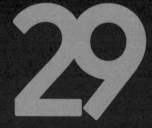

29

30

If you spend time online, why not create an inspiration board on Pinterest of the things that motivate and inspire you to be healthy?

31

Write down your long-term goal, then plan how you will achieve it in small steps. It will be less daunting this way.

32

A goal without a plan is just a wish.

33 Keep your expectations realistic. It's unlikely you'll look like an Olympic athlete even after you've lost a few pounds, but you can certainly aim to fit into that favourite pair of jeans.

Losing weight isn't a straight line. Your weight will fluctuate – particularly for women due to their monthly cycle – but don't panic. This is normal. **34**

35 Listen to your body and eat only when you're hungry – not when you're bored.

Next time you're tempted to snack, ask yourself if you want to eat an apple. If you're not hungry enough to eat an apple, you're probably not hungry.

Try not to view yourself as either 'on' or 'off' a diet. Viewing your healthy lifestyle as temporary will make it harder to form healthy habits for life.

Success is the sum of small efforts, repeated day in, day out.

39

When it comes to your diet, aim for
90 per cent fuel, 10 per cent fun.

40

Every day is a new chance to start taking care of yourself.

41

In two weeks, you'll feel it. In four weeks, you'll
see it. In eight weeks, you'll hear about it.

Put in the hard work now and enjoy the benefits for months and years to come.

Smaller adjustments to your eating habits will be more effective than drastic changes as they're things you will be likely to stick to.

44

Motivation gets you started,
habits keep you on track.

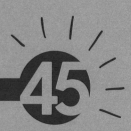

45

Remove temptation. Gather all of the sugary, processed
foods from your cupboards and donate it to a food
bank. Then restock your kitchen with healthy fare.

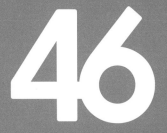

46

If you don't love it, don't eat it! If you're eating a 'meh' meal or dessert, put down your fork. There's no benefit to eating foods you're not *really* enjoying.

Avoid eating when you're distracted, such as snacking when you're watching TV or working at your desk. You're less likely to realise when you're full if you're not concentrating fully on your food.

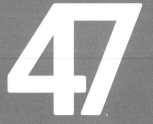

47

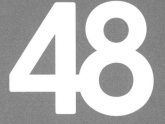

48

Burning off calories takes more work than you might think. If you find it hard to pick healthier options, remember, for instance, that a can of fizzy drink will take a few minutes to drink but up to an hour to burn off on the treadmill.

Use your hand as a portion guide for your main meal:

- **Protein:** the size of your palm.
- **Carbs and fruit:** your closed fist.
- **Nuts, cheese and other high-fat foods:** the size of your thumb.
- **Fats like butter and oil:** the size of one fingertip.
- **Vegetables:** the size of your outstretched hand.

50

Keep a food diary to help you become
aware of the things you eat.

51

In this diary, write down absolutely everything.
That includes a breath mint, a crisp from a
packet someone was sharing, or a second helping
of dinner, even if it was a small spoonful.

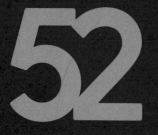

52

If you're more of a visual person, take photos of your food and keep track of it that way.

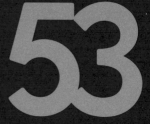

53

You may want to track your slimming journey visually by taking a photo of yourself every few weeks. You'll be able to see your progress, which can give your motivation a boost.

54

To reduce the temptation of second helpings, serve
yourself a portion, then put the leftovers out of
sight – you could even freeze them straight away
so you can't just go back for a little bit more.

55

Get familiar with the basics of nutrition. Understanding
what's in your food is the best way to learn how to
make informed decisions about what you eat.

56

A balanced diet will provide your body with all the sugar it needs for energy, so anything we consume in snacks, drinks, processed foods and sweet treats is usually surplus. So, for a healthy body you should aim to keep your sugar intake low, as this particularly is the energy that, when unused, turns to fat.

57

Sugar is not only found in baked goods and chocolate – it's present in most processed food. Check the labels when buying sauces, salad dressings, drinks and ready meals as there is often more sugar in them than you'd think.

58 Fruit can also be particularly high in sugar. Even though it's natural sugar, so better for you than the stuff in cakes and biscuits, you still shouldn't have too much.

59 Be wary of smoothies. They may seem like the healthy option, but they are the equivalent of eating several pieces of fruit at once, so the sugar content can be the same as eating a handful of sweets.

If you do want a smoothie then make your own, as this is a much healthier option. All you need to do is juice up a few of your favourite fruits in the blender and you're done!

If you're having a glass of fruit juice, dilute it with water.

Grapes, cherries, mangoes, figs and lychees are all fruits with a high sugar content, so be sparing with these fruits if you're snacking on them.

63

Strawberries, blackberries, raspberries and cranberries are all low in sugar, so add plenty of these juicy berries into your fruit salad and smoothies!

Yoghurt is another food that can be unhealthier than you might expect. Check the labels for their sugar content – even on the ones labelled as low fat – as some can contain as much as a chocolate bar. Anything with 6 g of sugar or less is a reasonable mark to aim for.

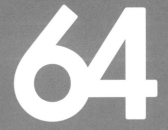

64

65

Many bottled, flavoured waters contain huge amounts of sugar – some more than fizzy drinks. If you crave more flavour in your H_2O, add it yourself with crushed mint, sliced ginger or sliced fruit.

If you're using sugar in recipes, try replacing it with honey or agave syrup – a natural and healthier alternative.

Dates can also be used as a substitute for sugar in some desserts. Puree them and add to recipes to make desserts and other treats healthier.

68

Make sure to include plenty of fibre in your diet. Not only does it keep your digestive system regular, but it helps to keep you feeling full for longer and prevent you from snacking. Fibre-rich foods include tangerines, bran cereal, oats, kidney beans and peas.

69

Another nutrient to be aware of when making food choices is fat, and the fact that not all of it is bad for you! Fat is vital for regulating your blood sugar levels and building cell walls, and it keeps you feeling full for longer.

70

Saturated fat is the one you want to avoid when you can. It's often found in meat and dairy products such as cheese and cream, in coconut oil, and in many processed foods such as cakes, biscuits, pizzas and crisps. High levels of saturated fat can lead to high cholesterol and a higher risk of heart disease.

71

A product is considered high in saturated fat if it contains more than 5 g of it per 100 g.

2

Unsaturated fat – often called 'good fat' – is the kind of fat that your body needs. It helps to keep you feeling full for a longer period, builds muscle and boosts your metabolic health, which makes it a vital part of your slimming journey. Find saturated fat in avocados, nuts, seeds, fish, olive oil and leafy vegetables.

3

The omega-3 fats from fortified foods or oily fish (such as tuna, salmon, sardines or mackerel) control hunger, reduce inflammation and keep your blood sugar steady.

Be wary about automatically choosing a low-fat product. In some instances, the fat has been replaced with sugar, so it could be just as unhealthy – if not more so – than the full fat version.

Download a food scanning app to make interpreting food labels easier. Simply scan the barcode of any food item and the app will use a traffic light colour code to show you how healthy the product is in terms of saturated fat, sugar and salt.

76

Just like fat, carbohydrates have had a lot of negative press, but they are your body's main source of energy, and they are vital to your health. The term 'carbohydrate' is very broad and covers three nutrients: sugar, starch and fibre. The most important thing is that the carbs you do eat are the right quality and quantity for your lifestyle.

Base your meals around starchy carbohydrates, such as bread, rice, potatoes and pasta, as these foods will release energy slowly over time and keep your blood sugar steady.

78

Choose complex brown carbs over white ones,
which are richer in fibre and nutrients. The same portion of
brown rice, brown bread and brown pasta will contain roughly
20–40 per cent fewer calories than its white counterpart.

79

**Don't overcook pasta. Your body absorbs
the sugar from al dente pasta more slowly, which means
you'll avoid spikes in blood sugar and feel fuller for longer.**

80 Cooled pasta is less fattening than just-cooked pasta and reheated pasta is less fattening still. This is because the body treats it more like a fibre than a starch and therefore absorbs fewer calories. The same is true of rice.

If you want a jacket potato for dinner but aren't sure which spud to choose, go for one that's approximately the same size as a travel-pack of tissues. A potato of this size will be about 100 calories. **81**

82

It's a myth that eating bread makes you fat. However, it isn't the most filling carbohydrate, so if you've had a bread-based lunch, for instance, you're more likely to need a snack later on. To stay fuller for longer, try packing a pasta or rice salad for lunch instead of a sandwich.

83

Sweet potatoes are great as a post-workout snack because they release their energy slowly and are high in fibre, which helps to satisfy that 'feed-me-now' hunger many people experience after they exercise.

84

Protein is the nutrient that helps your body to grow, build muscle tissue and repair itself. It also helps to stabilise your blood sugar and keep you feeling full. Protein is well known for being found in meat, fish, eggs and dairy products, but it can also be found in vegetable sources such as beans, pulses and nuts.

85

Protein-rich meals result in less hunger, more satisfaction and more fat being burned. Research has also found that people who eat meals that are high in protein generally eat 10 per cent less food per meal.

86

**The best meats to eat are low-fat
and protein-rich, such as fish or white meat.**

87

Not all meats are healthy sources of protein.
Red meats, especially processed red meat such as sausages,
ham, bacon or hot dogs, often contain a high quantity of
saturated fat and have been linked to heart disease, cancer,
diabetes and Alzheimer's. For the healthiest lifestyle,
consider reducing the amount of red meat you eat.

88

Spinach and kale have more iron per gram than beef, and you can get better quality protein from beans or soy products, so you do not miss out on vital nutrients by avoiding red meat.

However, there are ways you can make a healthy choice when it comes to red meat. It may be more expensive, but grass-fed beef is leaner and has fewer calories than regular beef. It also contains higher levels of omega-3 fatty acids, which reduce heart disease.

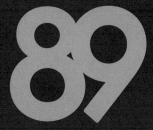

89

90

When it comes to a meat like pork, which can be fatty, choose a lean cut, such as tenderloin. This cut, on average, contains about the same number of calories as skinless chicken breast.

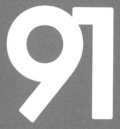

91

Ostrich meat has less fat than chicken or turkey and contains choline, a nutrient that helps with fat loss.

92

If you are eating meat with visible fat, simply cut the fat off your meat for an easy way to make your plate healthier.

93

Most people think that meat should be the main thing on their plate. Try thinking of it as a side to accompany your veggies and whole grains, or substituting it completely, as there are plenty of other protein sources available.

94

Cook bean-based meals to get a healthy dose of protein. Soy beans, lentils, kidney beans and white beans are all good legumes to pick. The average bean is also bursting with iron, magnesium and B vitamins, which are all top energy boosters.

95

Eggs, tofu, cottage cheese, broccoli and oats are all good sources of low-fat protein, and will help to fill you up and keep you satisfied throughout the day.

If you need a snack, eat a small handful of nuts – almonds or hazelnuts are a good choice. Their protein content means a small amount will help tide you over until your next meal.

97

Calcium-rich diets can aid weight loss,
so make sure you consume a healthy dose of milk
(or fortified alternative), seeds, leafy greens and canned fish.

98

For a healthy diet and a slimmer figurer, eating
vegetables is key! Vegetables are low in calories and high in
vitamins, minerals and fibre that your body needs, so you can eat
as much as you want and know that you're being good to yourself.

99 When you're planning your meals, include fruits and vegetables that are filling. Try artichokes, butternut squash, sweet potatoes, apples, cauliflower, berries, carrots, avocado, Brussels sprouts and pulses.

A simple way to get more veg into your diet is to create 'spaghetti' out of vegetables like courgettes, sweet potatoes, carrots and butternut squash with the help of a spiraliser. **100**

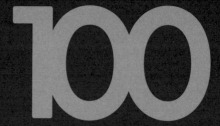

Another easy way to eat more vegetables is to substitute rice with cauliflower rice, which contains 85 per cent fewer calories than white rice. You can buy it ready-made or whip it up at home by grating cauliflower, or blitzing it in a food processor.

Potatoes are not the only food that can be mashed: try mashed cauliflower, turnip, swede or carrot as an alternative side dish.

103

Kale contains nutrients to combat belly fat and aid weight loss. If you don't like the regular kind, go for black kale or cavolo nero (aka dinosaur kale). It tastes sweeter and is more tender, but with all the same benefits.

104

When it comes to choosing your fruit, on the whole it's best to opt for fresh fruit when you can: 100 g of dried fruit can contain up to eight times more sugar and calories than the same amount of its fresh equivalent.

105

However, when enjoyed in moderation, dried fruit can be good for you. Prunes will lower cholesterol, regulate blood-sugar levels, increase satiety and help speed food through your digestive tract.

106

Cherry tomatoes are particularly low in calories, so you can eat them to your heart's content and pack a punch of healthy nutrients at the same time.

107

If you're looking for a healthy snack, eat a just-ripe banana. At this stage, they contain a source of resistant starch which the body digests more slowly, encouraging fullness.

108

Watermelon is 92 per cent water so, just like when you drink water, eating a portion of this fruit will make you feel fuller. Plus, not only is it juicy and delicious, but it can lower the risk of heart disease and your blood pressure too.

109

Eating half a grapefruit before meals has been
said to lower cholesterol and reduce visceral (belly)
fat due to its combination of phytochemicals – the
non-nutritive compounds in the plant – and vitamin C.

110

Kiwi fruits contain a sizeable amount of actinidin, an enzyme
that aids digestion by breaking down protein in the body.
Why not have one as a simple and healthy option for dessert?

For a trim waistline, always remember to eat breakfast. Not only does this meal refuel your body after a night of fasting and set you up for the day, helping your memory and concentration, and boosting your mood, but it also regulates your blood sugar, which means you're less likely to snack throughout the day too.

It's recommended that your breakfast contains 20–35 per cent of your daily calorie intake. If you consume 2,000 calories a day, your breakfast should be between 400 and 700 calories.

113

Studies have proven that the time of day you eat has more effect than what you eat, due to your body's internal clock. For the most efficient use of calories, eat your bigger meals for breakfast and lunch and a smaller meal for dinner.

114

A hearty breakfast with a blend of protein, fat and fibre is the way to go. For instance, nut butter on toast with banana will set you up for the day.

T15

For another healthy breakfast try oatmeal or porridge topped with a combination of nuts and berries.

T16

Cereal is another good breakfast option as it is often fortified with plenty of fibre and wholegrain. However, check the sugar content – it may contain more than you realise. Choose one that is high in fibre and low in sugar.

Vegetables often get overlooked at breakfast, but why not get the day off to a healthy, green start? Try spinach, mushrooms or avocado with scrambled eggs on toast.

If you're in a hurry and tend to eat your breakfast on the go, choose cereal bars that are sweetened with fruit rather than sugar.

Add a dollop of Greek yoghurt onto fruit, cereal or muesli as it contains plenty of protein and healthy fats, which will make you feel satisfied for longer.

120

If you have coffee with your breakfast, have a cup only after you've eaten. There is evidence to suggest that the caffeine empties your stomach more quickly if it's the first thing you consume; this means that your body doesn't absorb all the nutrients from your food, and you'll be hungry more quickly and tempted to snack.

121

Our bodies use 50 per cent more energy to digest whole food compared with processed foods, meaning we only take in half of the calories from whole foods. Eating processed food is therefore effectively giving you twice the number of calories as the equivalent from whole foods. Cut down on the processed stuff wherever you can.

122

You're more likely to stick to making a healthy lifestyle a habit if you're enjoying it, so be adventurous with healthy food and find things you love!

123

If you need some inspiration, turn to a recipe book. There are plenty available that cater to all tastes and budgets – browse your bookshop or a local library to find one that suits you.

124

The best way to know exactly what you're
eating is to don your apron and make your meals from scratch.
Healthy home-made meals can be as simple or complex as
you want them to be, so whatever your schedule or your
ability in the kitchen there'll be something you can cook.

125

For every meal, aim for your plate to contain
roughly one quarter slow-release carbs, one quarter
protein, and one half vegetables.

126

Popcorn is a whole grain, so it can be good for you in small portions and will help maintain a healthy gut. Try sprinkling cinnamon or curry powder over it (instead of butter, sugar or salt) for a healthy snack.

127

Eat a handful of fennel seeds after a meal to alleviate gas and reduce bloating.

128

Keep each snack to 125 calories or less. Try these: a hard-boiled egg, nut butter spread on a rice cake, a fig bar, two tablespoons of hummus on half a pitta or three tablespoons of raisins.

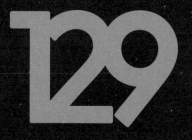

129

Whip up this simple, healthy snack: mix 80 g chopped dates, 80 g nut butter and 50 g rolled oats, then shape them into balls, put in an airtight container in a cool place and wait for them to harden.

Pistachios contain a winning combo of healthy fats, fibre and protein to keep you satisfied throughout the day. The fact that you have to deshell them also helps you to banish mindless snacking.

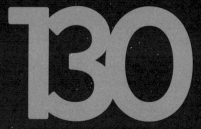

130

Freeze grapes for a fruity treat that feels like eating an ice lolly.

Jazz up an apple by baking it, then dolloping on 1 tbsp of low-fat yoghurt and a sprinkling of cinnamon.

Freeze tubes of yoghurts and eat instead of an ice cream. Fro-yo a go-go!

134

Bake your own vegetable crisps with sliced parsnips, carrots, sweet potatoes, beetroot or kale and a light drizzle of olive oil: healthier and more flavoursome than salty, processed crisps.

135

Snack on a small portion of Edam cheese.
With a 20-gram portion approximately 70 calories,
it's the perfect snack to provide you with some
filling protein without being too unhealthy.

136

Chop up a pitta bread and bake to form pitta chips. Use them as an alternative to tortilla chips when eating guacamole, salsa and other dips.

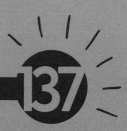

137

Pumpkin seeds are high in fibre and protein, so they leave you feeling fuller for longer. Blend them with basil, garlic and Parmesan cheese to make pesto, or toast them and sprinkle onto salads.

138

Tofu is packed with protein and contains just 80 calories per serving. It works particularly well marinated and added to stir-fries or curries.

139

Coconuts provide sugar for energy while its healthy fat means your body digests it slowly. Sprinkle unsweetened flakes over cereal or use low-fat coconut milk in a curry to prevent hunger and steady your blood-sugar levels.

140

Eat cashew butter instead of peanut butter. It contains less sugar and fewer additives and calories.

141

Instead of spaghetti, eat spaghetti squash. This vegetable with flesh that resembles spaghetti in look, taste and texture has just 31 calories per 100 g compared with pasta's 158.

142

Steam or stir-fry veggies rather than boiling them (which removes vital nutrients).

143

If a recipe calls for mayonnaise, substitute half the amount with plain yoghurt to reduce the calorie count.

144

Swap creamy dips for healthy, fresh salsa. Eat it with batons of veggies rather than crisps and you'll still get that satisfying crunch.

145

Use turkey or vegetarian mince in your Bolognese sauce for a less fattening alternative to beef mince.

146

If you stick to using beef mince, make sure it's lean, with five per cent or less fat.

147

Fry things using a cooking spray, rather than in oil or butter.

148

If you're baking cookies, use vegetable oil or apple sauce instead of butter.

149

Choose dark chocolate instead of milk or white. It contains less sugar than other varieties of chocolate, and the pure cocoa butter it's made from means it's digested more slowly, so it staves off hunger. It's also a great source of vitamin C, antioxidants and fibre.

150

You don't have to stop going out for meals to live a healthy lifestyle – it's just down to making the right choices. If you're having Italian, for example, go for a pasta dish with a tomato-based sauce rather than a creamy carbonara.

151 Have a low-calorie starter such as a salad or non-creamy soup as this will help to prevent overeating during your main course and will be healthier than a dessert.

152 Before you eat out at a restaurant, look at the menu online first. You'll be able to research the nutritional information before you dine in order to make wise choices.

153 If you're having a Chinese takeaway, avoid ordering anything described as 'crispy' – this means fried.

154

When ordering a coffee, avoid anything with cream, which contains a lot of fat, and any syrup flavourings as these are high in sugar. You could also opt for skimmed or non-dairy milk.

155

If you treat yourself to sweets or chocolates, choose wrapped versions. A study found that people ate 30 per cent less if they had to unwrap what they ate first.

156

If you want chips, choose ones that have been baked rather than fried.

157

Don't be deceived by the name; if you're choosing between chunky chips and skinny fries, go for the former. Chunky fries contain less fat because they soak up less oil while cooking.

158

Swap salt for healthier flavourings, such as herbs, spices, lemon, mustard, pepper or chilli.

159

Blot your pizza with a piece of kitchen towel
to soak up any excess oil and grease.

160

Grill or roast food instead of frying it in lots of oil.

161

Have sorbet instead of ice cream. Better yet, make your
own! Freeze banana chunks and then blend with cinnamon,
cocoa powder or berries for a healthy but delicious dessert.

162

If you do have ice cream, an easy way to make your treat that little bit better for you is to eat from a cup rather than a cone.

163

Tweak your treat! Instead of a chocolate-chip muffin, get a carrot or raisin one.

164

Buy tinned goods (tuna, olives, fruits and vegetables) packed in water rather than oil or syrup.

165

Instead of using two slices of bread for your sandwich, just use one and have an open sandwich. Add plenty of toppings to pack in flavour and extra nutrients.

166

When baking sweet treats, look for recipes that use vegetables. Avocado, courgette and beetroot all make great cake bases and don't taste like you're eating veggies, promise!

167

Fruits and veg can sometimes be affected by pesticides that can decrease your metabolism and make losing weight harder. Try buying organic foods and see if it makes a difference to how you feel.

168

Base your meals around what's seasonal and plentiful in the shops. This will help to make it easier to include vegetables – and a wide range of them – in your diet.

169

Buy ready-cut vegetables to save on chopping, slicing and dicing. The easier you make it on yourself to make a quick and healthy meal, the better.

170

Beware of the word 'low'. Often if food is deemed low in something (like carbs), it's often high in something else (like fat).

Your body's metabolism is regulated by the thyroid gland, so keep yours healthy by including plenty of vitamin A and D in your diet; drink herbal teas and eat high-fibre foods like apples, almonds and chickpeas.

There is some evidence to suggest that eating foods that contain chilli can help you lose weight, as the spiciness increases your heart rate and boosts your metabolism.

173

Capsaicin – the thing that makes chillies hot – also suppresses appetite, so add chillies to casseroles, soups and stir-fries to feel full on smaller portion sizes.

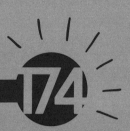

174

Keep a bag of frozen veg in your freezer so you can inject a healthy kick into meals easily if you haven't had time to buy fresh produce.

T75

Pad out your meals with water-rich vegetables like peppers, courgettes, tomatoes and lettuce.

T76

Eat tabbouleh. The bulgur wheat is packed with protein and fibre to crush hunger pangs, and the olive oil increases levels of serotonin, which is linked to satiety.

T77

Evidence suggests that acetic acid, the main component of vinegar, helps to reduce blood pressure and the formation of fat – so eat vinegar-based salad dressings and pickled veg.

178

Cinnamon has been shown to help reduce belly fat by stabilising blood-sugar levels and controlling appetite. Sprinkle some on your porridge or into a smoothie.

179

Add turmeric to your stir-fry, latte or breakfast. It contains curcumin, which is said to suppress the growth of fat tissue and increase fat burning.

180

Ginger can help you slim down for a number of reasons: it's a natural appetite suppressant, it lowers cholesterol, it aids digestion and it boosts metabolism. Try including a ginger tea in your diet.

Drink green tea. It contains a powerful antioxidant that raises your metabolic rate, burns calories and increases the speed at which your body uses fat. It also contains the amino acid theanine, which promotes calmness, so it helps you to both look and feel great!

181

182

Try pu-erh tea – a fermented Chinese brew
that is said to shrink fat cells in the body.

183

Drink oolong, or 'black dragon': a Chinese tea
packed with nutrients that boost the body's ability
to metabolise fat, which helps with weight loss.

184

Drinking lemon water – hot or cold – can aid weight loss by
boosting your metabolism, helping digestion and keeping your appetite at bay.
It will also cleanse your liver, boost your immune system and firm your skin.

185

When you have a craving for a particular food, it usually means your body is trying to tell you something. Rather than giving in to the craving and eating the sweet/salty/crunchy snack, or trying to ignore your body completely, listen to it and try out a healthy alternative to satisfy the itch.

186

If you're craving something salty, try having a handful of dry-roasted nuts, which will give you the salty kick you're after with plenty of healthy fats and protein too. Alternatively, have a handful of olives.

187

Reduce the likelihood of salt cravings by staying hydrated and drinking plenty of water throughout the day.

188

If you feel the need for something sweet, it probably means your blood sugar is low. Turn to the fruit bowl and satisfy the need for sweetness with natural sugar, rather than refined sugar. Try a kiwi, a banana, or a handful of cherries or grapes.

189

If what you really want is something crunchy, have a few sticks of celery instead of a packet of crisps.

190

If you're craving bread it could mean that your body is low on nitrogen. You can restore the balance in a healthy way by eating a handful of protein-rich nuts, seeds or legumes such as chickpeas.

191

A cheese craving could mean that your body is low on essential fatty acids, so try having a handful of walnuts or chia seeds to curb it.

192

Feeling the need for cheese could also mean that you're not getting enough calcium. Green vegetables such as kale, broccoli and spinach can give you a top-up, as can salmon, sardines and white beans.

193

Chromium is essential in the body to help metabolise fats and carbohydrates, and not having enough of it is sometimes the reason that we crave white bread and pasta. Apples, grapes, broccoli, tomatoes and sweet potatoes are all good sources of chromium to fill up on instead.

194

If you want to know more about the foods that
work best for you, speak to a nutritional therapist.
They can evaluate your lifestyle and come up with
a nutrition plan to help you stay healthy.

195

Take a vitamin D supplement. If you have a low level of this
'sunshine vitamin', you may store more fat, and your brain will
release hunger-signalling hormones, tempting you to snack.

196

If you have a large plate or bowl it's easy to eat more than you need, as they make a normal serving of food look smaller than it is. To help keep your sense of perspective, serve your meals on a smaller plate.

197

Use measuring scales and cups to portion out your food and ensure you're only eating one serving.

198

Portion out snacks in small bags or reusable boxes to take to work. You'll be less likely to pop to the vending machine or cafe.

199

The colour blue is thought to be an appetite suppressant, so you could serve food on blue plates or use a blue tablecloth and cutlery while you eat.

200

Try to minimise the colours red, orange or yellow in the area where you're dining. Studies have found that they can encourage overeating.

201

Chewing your food for longer will help you feel fuller more quickly, so you'll eat less.

202

Try not to eat standing in front of the fridge. If you're eating mindlessly you're more likely to consume calories you don't need.

203

If you have a snack from a larger bag, portion it out before you start eating. For instance, when eating crisps, instead of munching straight from the bag, empty a small serving into a bowl. When they're gone, they're gone.

204

Get into the habit of simply declining sugary snacks when they're offered around (especially if they're of the biscuit/cake variety!). This is an easy way to reduce your intake of empty calories in day-to-day life.

205

Keep a healthy snack in your bag – perhaps some (unsalted) nuts – so you can refuel on the go, rather than grabbing something sugar-laden when you feel peckish.

206

Learn your body's signals. When your stomach is full, it pushes against the diaphragm and you'll sigh. This is your body saying, 'Enough'.

207

Drink water before and during your meals to help fill you up more.

208

If plain water bores you, infuse it with fruits, herbs and veggies. How about lemon and mint, cucumber and blueberry, or strawberry and basil?

Drinking water throughout the day helps to reduce bloating. Aim for around two litres a day.

209

210

A treat doesn't have to be something that you eat. Spoil yourself with a bubble bath, a good book or an engrossing film instead.

211

Plan and prepare a few of these non-edible treats in advance. Next time you have the urge to reach for the biscuits, your non-edible rewards will already be there waiting for you, and will give you the boost that you need.

212

Unfortunately, calories at the weekend DO count! Try not to undo all your midweek hard work by 'rewarding yourself' come Friday evening.

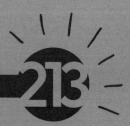

213

Don't be tempted to skip meals. Doing this causes your blood sugar levels to plummet and you'll crave a sugary snack.

214

Plan your meals in advance – maybe for a week,
or for however long you go between shopping trips –
so you can create healthy, tasty meals to look forward to.

215

At the beginning of each day, decide what you're
going to eat. Three meals and two snacks is a sensible way to go.
When you know exactly when your next snack/meal is coming
it can help to reduce the amount you think or worry about it.

216

Planning can also help curb your hunger levels. If you stick to an eating schedule and plan meals and snacks at the same time each day, your body will learn to anticipate food times and adapt hormone cycles accordingly.

Make meal planning easier by batch-cooking healthy dinners and freezing leftovers so that they are readily available.

217

218

Write a list before you go to the supermarket to avoid impulse buys.

219

Shop online to avoid having to walk past tempting treats altogether.

220

Use the self-checkout till. According to one study, impulse buys dropped by around 32 per cent for women and 17 per cent for men when they did this.

Use a trolley rather than a basket at the supermarket and you are more likely to make informed food choices. If you are lugging around a heavy basket and want to get to the check-out as soon as possible, reading food labels often goes out the window.

Be aware of the calorie content in alcohol. A large glass of wine contains the same number of calories as a doughnut, and a pint of lager is the equivalent to a large slice of pizza.

223

Alcohol encourages fluid retention and increases fatty deposits in the thighs, stomach, arms and bum. Booze can also cause bloating, so for optimum health and a slim figure, reduce the amount you drink.

224

If you are drinking, choose a half pint or a small glass of alcohol and drink it slowly to make it last – you won't feel deprived but you will halve the number of calories you drink.

225

Try to avoid getting drunk. Research has shown that the neurons in your brain that provoke hunger are activated by alcohol (that explains the lure of the 2 a.m. kebab...).

226

When you drink alcohol, you're also more sensitive to the aroma of food, which means you're less likely to resist something tempting or indulgent.

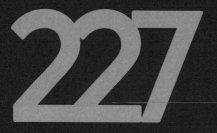

227

Although alcohol will never be a healthy drink, there are healthier choices you can make. Pinot noir contains the highest level of resveratrol among all the wines. Resveratrol is a plant component found in the skin of red grapes, among other plants, and evidence suggests that it can encourage fat loss.

Craft beer also typically contains lots of nutrients, soluble fibre, B vitamins, antioxidants and silicon, so in some ways it is a healthier option than other beers. However, it does also contain twice the alcohol and calories of regular beer, so choose carefully and be sure not to overindulge.

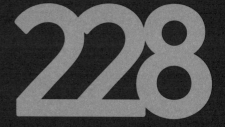

228

229

Use a tall, thin glass rather than a short, squat one.
Research has shown that people drink 25–30 per cent
less this way as the mind thinks 'taller' equals 'more'.

230

Make your goal a lifetime eating plan, not a diet.

231

Get the people you frequently dine with on board with
your healthy eating habits. This will help to limit situations
in which you feel social pressure to eat unhealthily.

232

Try dimming the lights before you eat your meal.
Research has shown that you'll eat less.

233

Eat while listening to soft music. Studies show that you'll
savour your food more and won't eat as quickly. As well as this
helping you to feel full, you'll also enjoy your food more!

234

Sit down to eat any meals or snacks. Research has shown that we eat more quickly when we're standing up, often resulting in overeating and consuming more calories.

235

When you eat your dinner, do so mindfully, chewing each mouthful and savouring all the flavours and textures – studies show this makes you feel more satisfied and helps you appreciate your food more.

236

It takes about 20 minutes for feelings of fullness to reach your brain, so eat slowly to allow you to get the message before you overeat. Taking your time will also increase your feelings of satiety.

237

If you have trouble remembering to eat slowly, hold your knife and fork in the opposite hands to usual to slow you down.

238

Put down your fork between each mouthful to encourage you to eat at a more leisurely pace.

239

Eat desserts with a teaspoon to savour the taste for longer and encourage you to eat more slowly.

240

Chat more while you're eating. You won't eat so quickly and you'll entertain your dining companion too.

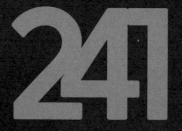

241

If you're not already proficient at using chopsticks, try using a pair to help you eat more slowly.

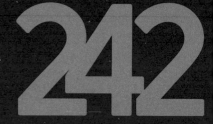

242

Retrain yourself to only eat until you are 80 per cent full – a Japanese practice called *hara hachi bu*. By stopping eating when you are no longer hungry, instead of when you are completely full, your stomach can process the food more efficiently and is not at risk of being stretched.

243

Stress can slow down your body's metabolism,
causing poor digestion, and increase cortisol levels,
which can ultimately increase body fat.

244

A good way to reduce stress is to practice calming
breathing techniques. If you feel tense, take a few minutes
on your own. Sit somewhere comfortable and quiet,
and breathe in through your nose slowly and deeply.
Hold your breath for a few seconds, and exhale slowly
through your mouth. Repeat until you feel calm.

245

Caffeine, alcohol and nicotine are all substances that can exacerbate feelings of stress. Try reducing your intake for a calmer mind and healthier body.

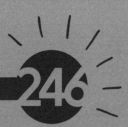

246

Exercise is one of the best stress busters there is. It's an opportunity for you to release your pent-up energy, and exercise triggers endorphins, the feel-good chemicals in your brain, improving your mood.

247

Try aromatherapy to help relieve symptoms of stress. Light a scented candle or take a bubble bath with a few drops of essential oil.

248

The best way to combat stress is to get to the root of it and tackle the cause rather than the symptom. If you regularly find yourself feeling stressed, identify why this might be. Is it a particular person, place or activity that's causing you to feel this way?

249

If you struggle with emotional eating, know that you are not alone – many people deal with this problem. Most importantly, don't beat yourself up about it. Instead, focus on what you can do to avoid it in the future.

250

Identify what your triggers are. Is it a particular person, place or event? For instance, if stress at work is a trigger, bring a healthy, crunchy snack with you next time you have a big meeting coming up, and know that you can eat that without any of the ill effects of unhealthy food.

251

Eating can be a way to numb the discomfort of painful emotions or distract ourselves from them. Next time you are feeling angry, sad, guilty, confused, or any other emotion that makes you want to eat, sit for a few minutes and let yourself feel those emotions instead of pushing them away. Through this you can often find what it is you really want or need.

252

If you tend to want to eat when you're feeling sad, try calling a friend next time you sense an episode coming on. Whether you talk to them about your immediate feelings or chat about something else entirely, seeking support from loved ones can often help to make you feel better.

253

If you eat to relieve stress, look into alternative ways to release it. Exercise such as running or boxing can be effective, but some non-active options to try are breathing exercises, listening to loud music, singing or shouting loudly, or something proactive such as tidying up or organising. When you feel the urge to eat emotionally, ground your body and mind.

254

Focus on the objects around you – notice their appearance, texture, small details – and take a few minutes to breathe. Let any panic or frenzied feelings pass. This will help you to get out of your head and back into the present.

255

Aim to get around eight hours of sleep a night. This will help to reduce your levels of the hunger hormone, ghrelin.

256

Not getting enough sleep increases the stress hormone cortisol. In turn, this encourages you to overeat to refuel after dealing with pressure and worry.

257

Lack of sleep hinders impulse control, which means you're more likely to give in to cravings and reach for unhealthy foods.

258

Eat almonds, oats, lettuce, turkey and potatoes to increase your production of melatonin, the hormone that helps you sleep.

Bananas have been called 'nature's sleeping pill' as the potassium and magnesium they contain helps to relax nerves and muscles, and encourages a serene slumber.

259

260

Don't eat anything substantial for two to three hours before bedtime. This will help you avoid insomnia and heartburn, and allows your body to fall into deep sleep.

There is also evidence to suggest that eating food
late at night means you're more likely to gain weight,
so avoid snacking after you've finished your dinner.

Eating a tablespoon of raw honey an hour before
bed can help keep your blood sugar stable overnight,
to fuel the liver and improve sleep.

Put screens away at least half an hour before bed,
so that the blue light they emit doesn't harm your sleep.

264

Download an app to reduce the amount of blue
light that's emitted from your phone or tablet screen.
Some devices have this feature built in – if yours does, enable it.

265

Have a warm shower or bath before bed.
As your body cools down it also slows down – your heart
and breathing rates begin to drop, for instance, and your
digestion slows. This makes it easier for us to fall asleep.

266

Brush your teeth after you've eaten. It will take away the taste of food and stop you craving more, and afterwards you won't want to ruin your mouth's minty freshness.

267

Avoid the bread basket in restaurants or nibbles laid out on the table. Small amounts of food still add up to extra calories and are harder to keep track of!

268

Set yourself achievable goals to help you to get into healthy eating habits. For instance, for one week, aim to have porridge for breakfast instead of sugary cereal.

269

Have a 'slimming buddy'. Meet regularly to check in about your progress and offer each other encouragement.

Research has shown that people who share their slimming goals and progress on social media have more chance of successful weight loss. So, get sharing!

270

271 Have more sex. Not only can the average steamy session burn up to 100 calories, the endorphins released during an orgasm are said to suppress your appetite.

272 Create an end-of-meal habit (that doesn't involve eating dessert). Go for a walk, read the news, do the dishes... anything to send a message to your brain that eating is over.

273 Another example could be lighting a candle when you sit down for dinner. When you've eaten all you need to, blow it out.

274

Replace your snacking rituals with other activities. For instance, if you always go to the kitchen after coming home, play some music instead.

275

Eat three fewer bites than you intended to of every meal. This way, you're likely to reduce your calorie intake by about 100 calories a day without much extra effort.

276

Once you've lost weight, give away your clothes that are now too big. Having to buy a whole new wardrobe if you gain weight again will be a good incentive to stay slim.

277

Late-evening snacking significantly increases the number of calories you eat a day. Create a routine to 'close your kitchen' after dinner – do the dishes, turn out the light and close the door.

278

When you eat in a restaurant you're more likely to eat a large portion (and foods that are high in fat), so try to eat at home more than you eat out.

279

When you're ordering food that offers different portion sizes, ask for the smallest portion rather than the regular or large. Restaurants and cafes tend to offer large portions anyway, so with their smallest serving you'll have enough food without the needless extra.

280

Think of high-calorie treats in a different way. Instead of a bowl of ice cream with a spoonful of fruit, have a bowl of fruit with a spoonful of ice cream.

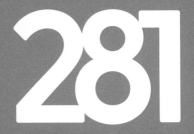

281
Instead of pouring the dressing onto your salad, empty it into a dish and then dip your empty fork into it, before spearing your lettuce. This way you get all of the flavour and fewer calories.

Many recipes suggest topping meals with cheese to serve – a simple way to be healthier is just to skip this step! The meal you've made will still be delicious but without the extra fat.

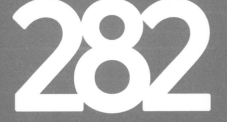

282

283
If you can't resist a dessert, share one!

284

You don't need to turn down the slice of birthday cake, but if you scrape the icing off, it will help to reduce the amount of sugar you eat.

285

Dab vanilla extract on your wrists or light a vanilla-scented candle. It's thought that the whiff of vanilla leads to fewer cravings, particularly for sweet treats.

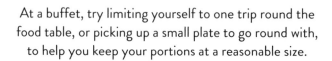

286

At a buffet, try limiting yourself to one trip round the food table, or picking up a small plate to go round with, to help you keep your portions at a reasonable size.

287

If you think you're hungry, have a glass
of water first and wait for 15 minutes.
Then see if you still fancy a snack.

288

Don't sit near the 'treat table' at work. If you can't
move your desk, ask if you can move the goodies to
a different place. Out of sight, out of mind.

289

If you're heading to the fridge, or the snack cupboard, take a
detour via your laptop, or busy yourself with that one job that you've been meaning
to do for weeks. It's quite possible you'll forget that you even wanted a snack.

290 Tell others about your plans to eat well. Letting people know allows them to be considerate and not offer you sweet treats, and they can offer you encouragement if you're ever feeling low or unmotivated.

291 Chewing gum can satisfy your sweet cravings and manage hunger. Just make it the sugar-free variety.

292 If you find you have the urge to nibble as you're making dinner, chop up an extra carrot to crunch on while you cook.

293

The average food craving lasts for about
15 minutes, so wait it out and see if it passes.

294

Standing burns more calories than sitting. Why not stand
up while you're watching TV, or playing on your phone?

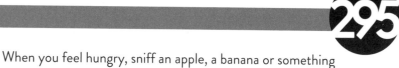

295

When you feel hungry, sniff an apple, a banana or something
peppermint-flavoured and your brain will be tricked into
thinking you're actually eating what you're smelling.

296

Every time you shop for food, make one positive swap. If you always buy cookies, buy something healthy you've never tried before instead, like a new type of fruit or vegetable.

297

Don't allow an indulgent meal break you out of good habits. It's easy to slip into the mindset that says, 'I've already eaten something bad, so I may as well eat more...' But that's not how your body works!

298 Store biscuits and other treats in an inconvenient place – in a tin, on a high shelf. If they're a hassle to get to, you may think twice about eating them.

299 Try peeling, chopping or segmenting your healthy snack the night before or in the morning before you leave the house. This makes it much easier for you to snack on something healthy on a whim.

300 Exercise is a key part of slimming and also important in maintaining your weight. So, if you want to slim down, get active!

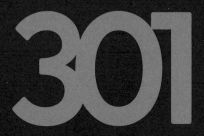

301

When it comes to exercise, don't go too fast too soon. If you try something too hard, or you begin a regime that you can't realistically keep up, you'll become discouraged and you're more likely to quit. The trick is to start slowly and gradually increase the intensity of your training.

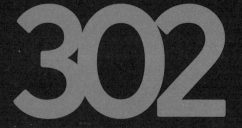

302

Don't be discouraged if you put on weight at first. As you work out, you're going to convert fat to muscle, which will make you fitter, firmer and – yes – slightly heavier. Gauge your progress by how you feel, rather than by what the scales say.

303

In terms of how well it measures your health, your weight on its own is an arbitrary figure: the same weight will be different on everyone depending on their age, gender, height and body type. Instead, calculate your body mass index (BMI) to work out the ideal healthy weight for you, as this takes your age, height and gender into account. There are calculators online that can do this for you.

304

Factor exercise into your daily routine. Even going for a walk during your lunch break will get your blood pumping and benefit you.

305

Wear an activity tracker around your wrist to note your progress. Among other things, it can record the number of steps you've taken, calories burned, distance travelled and your quality of sleep.

306

When you've done your exercise for the day, resist the temptation to reward yourself with an unhealthy snack!

307

To refuel healthily after a workout, opt for a banana, an apple, a couple of dates, or sweet potatoes.

308

Muscles burn more calories than fat, so include weight training in your fitness plans. If you develop your muscles your body can naturally burn up to 40 per cent more calories a day without doing a thing.

309

Whatever kind of exercise you're doing, whether it's running, swimming, dancing, walking, playing a sport, or strength training, make sure you warm up before you start and cool down once you've finished. This will help to prevent injury and keep your body strong.

310

A brisk walk or jogging on the spot are both good warm-ups. The aim is to increase your heart rate steadily; this way your blood will take more oxygen and glucose to your muscles, which can increase your physical performance and burn more calories.

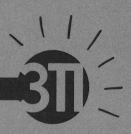

311

High-intensity sprinting burns fat. This involves running as fast and hard as possible for 30 seconds to a minute, followed by 4 minutes of a light jog. This cycle is repeated four or five times. It will elevate your heart rate and put your body into an 'oxygen debt', which allows you to burn fat hours after your workout finishes.

312

Work squats into your daily routine. This simple exercise will increase your body's strength and muscle, reduce cellulite, improve your circulation, flexibility and posture, tone your legs and bum – and you'll burn fat, too!

313

If you find doing squats or running on the treadmill boring, try working out to your favourite TV programme – it'll make the time go quicker and is less time spent sitting on the couch: win–win!

314

Take the stairs instead of the lift to add a quick burst of activity into your day.

315

Park further away than you need to so you can get your steps in, or get off the bus one stop early.

316

Do squats or star jumps in the kitchen while you wait for the kettle to boil, or for food to cook. Even raising your heart rate for a few minutes at a time benefits your body.

317

Dance like no one is watching – an energetic dance session for just 15 minutes can burn up to 100 calories.

318

If you own a bike, cycle rather than drive wherever possible.

319

Chores can be good for you – even low-intensity household activities like cleaning will burn fat. For instance, scrubbing for half an hour could burn about 120 calories.

320

Walk the dog, or ask if you can walk a friend or neighbour's if you don't have one. It's great exercise and it's a stressbuster too!

321

Don't be afraid to multitask. If you're on the phone, pick up a hand weight with your other arm and pump some iron. It needn't be a real weight either – anything heavy (a full water bottle, a bag of sugar) will do.

322

If you're standing waiting for the bus or in a queue, squeeze
your abs in tight and hold for a count of ten, then slowly
release as you exhale. Do ten repetitions, three times. This
is an easy way to give your core a covert mini workout.

323

Does your day often run away with you?
Exercise first thing in the morning before your
to-do list overtakes your good intentions.

324

If the gym's not your thing, try swimming, tennis, belly dancing... any exercise that you'll look forward to doing.

325

Put energy into your walk; swing your arms a little more, or take bigger strides. Moving more in little ways all adds up to make a difference.

326

Burn ten calories before you've even got out of bed. When you wake up, sit up slowly without using your hands. Keep your legs straight out and lean forward until you feel a gentle stretch in your hamstrings and back. Hold, then lower yourself back to the bed, using your stomach muscles. Do this three times.

327

Burn a further ten calories – and develop your core – while brushing your teeth. Do this by standing on one leg and alternating every 30 seconds.

328

Yoga is excellent exercise for building muscle which, in turn, boosts metabolism. It also encourages mindfulness, which will help you tune in to your body.

Walking for weight loss is great; Nordic walking is even better. This sport involves using poles to help you walk, which utilises the muscles in your shoulders, arms and torso as well as your legs, making your walk a full-body workout.

329

330

While you're stuck in traffic or sitting at your desk, clench your bum muscles for a count of ten, then release. Do this 15 times throughout the day.

331

Walk while you talk. Pacing about or going for a stroll while you're on the phone will burn calories when you'd otherwise be sitting.

332

At work use a toilet or printer on a different floor to encourage you to walk more. Every bit of movement in your day makes a difference.

333

When you're running errands or doing your weekly shop, wear a backpack with a bag of sugar (or something heavier) inside. You'll increase resistance and burn calories without even trying.

334

Tone your calves while making a cup of tea. While you're waiting for the kettle to boil, stand on the balls of your feet and raise yourself up slowly, then come back down again. Repeat the exercise until you feel the effects (or until your tea has brewed!).

335

Throwing a Frisbee or kicking a ball around for half an hour with a friend is not only fun, but it can burn up to 100 calories.

336

Do wall push-ups. Place your hands wide against a wall at shoulder height and take two steps back so you're at an angle and your weight is on your toes. Do three sets of ten push-ups.

337

While sitting at your desk, extend your right leg until it's level with your hip, then slowly lower it. Repeat ten times and swap legs. Hello, toned thighs!

338

Don't mix cardio and weight training in the same session – alternate between them instead. Your workouts will have more impact and long-term benefits if you keep them separate, as you will be too fatigued from one to reap any benefits from the other when combined.

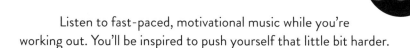

339

Listen to fast-paced, motivational music while you're
working out. You'll be inspired to push yourself that little bit harder.

340

Do burpees. They increase heart rate, work your legs,
arms and abs, and seriously blitz calories. If you're unsure of how to
do them, look up a video tutorial to make sure you're doing them correctly.

341

Exercise with a friend so you can help to spur each other on.

342

Consider a session with a personal trainer – they will be able to tailor a workout programme to your current fitness level and goal.

343

Aim to break a sweat every day, even if it's just for a few minutes. Regular exercise, little and often, will do wonders for your body.

344

The plank is an amazing exercise to slim your waistline, as well as work on your core. Begin by holding it for a few seconds and see if you can increase the length of time you can hold the position over the course of a month.

345

If you're struggling to lose weight despite eating healthily and exercising, talk to your doctor. As well as providing extra information on a healthy lifestyle, they can help to determine whether there are any underlying problems that are affecting your weight, such as hormone imbalances.

346

If your goal is to do 20 sit-ups, do 20 sit-ups. If you give up after 10, you're only cheating yourself.

347

If you feel like skipping an exercise session, ask yourself whether you will regret it if you do.

348

Plan when you will exercise each week and put it in your diary. Treat each allotment as an important appointment that can't be rescheduled or cancelled.

349

If you're determined and you keep working hard, you will see results.

350

Everyone who exercises regularly was once a beginner.

351

Remember, there are 21 meals in a week. If one goes awry, focus on the other 20.

352

The weight didn't go on overnight and it won't come off overnight. But keep going and it *will* come off.

353

Do the very best that you can today.

354

You may not be there yet but you are closer than you were yesterday.

If you don't want to start again, don't give up.

355

356

One salad won't make you thin, just like one cake doesn't make you fat. It takes time to change.

357

Focus on what you *are* eating
rather than what you're *not*.

358

Everything in moderation is the key to success.

359

Visualise how you'll look and feel when you reach your
goal – and hold on to that feeling whenever you need a boost.

360

Don't compare yourself to others. Remember, this is your slimming journey and your body, so take it at your own pace.

361

If you can make it through one day, you can make it through another.

362

Bin the guilt. If you fall off the wagon, don't beat yourself up. Just climb back on.

Aim for progress, not perfection.

Use your mind to change your body.

Believe in yourself!
If you can imagine it, you can do it.

If you're interested in finding out more about our books, find us on Facebook at **Summersdale Publishers** and follow us on Twitter at **@Summersdale**.

www.summersdale.com